1

The Best Darn CFS, Fibromyalgia and Adrenal Fatigue Book!

Studies on Syndromes of Pain, Tiredness and Hypoadrenia

By: James M. Lowrance © 2010

TABLE OF CONTENTS:

CHAPTER ONE

Common Symptoms of Chronic Fatigue Syndrome

A Medically Recognized Illness

According to medical research and sources, Chronic Fatigue Syndrome (CFS) is characterized by its main symptom of "fatigue" not explained by another existing illness.
In order for severe, chronic fatigue to be considered as a possibility for being caused by CFS, it must be experienced for at least six months, with no significant relief during any of this time period. It is also described by medical criteria (for diagnosis) as not being relieved by sleep or rest.

People suffering CFS will find that sleep does not refresh them, even when they get adequate or more-than adequate amounts of sleep (eight hours or more). This symptom of severe, chronic fatigue is the major, characterizing feature of CFS, including post exertional malaise (intolerance to physical exercise and exertion).

Joint and Muscle Pain

People with CFS will find that they have joint and muscle aches that are very concerning and somewhat disabling, but the joints and muscles will not swell or exhibit redness around them (as happens with different types of arthritis). These joint and muscle aches will be mild to moderate and may also cause stiffness and slightly reduced mobility.

The body aches often resemble those experienced when a person has the flu. With some CFS patients, this symptom is intermittent and with others, it is continual.

If a patient has more severe and widespread body pain, along with "tender points," which are small areas where the muscle attaches to joints that are very tender to finger-point pressure, this can indicate "Fibromyalgia Syndrome" (FMS) rather than Chronic Fatigue Syndrome. These two syndromes have been found to have 75% crossover similarities.

Swollen Lymph Nodes

According to the U.S. Centers for Disease Control (CDC), "swollen lymph nodes" are also a major symptom of CFS. Those that become swollen are commonly located in the neck, just under the tonsil area on both sides, with swelling being detectable to the touch (palpation) and are also referred to as glands ("nodes" is the correct term). Lymph nodes under the armpits are also commonly found to be swollen with cases of CFS.

Medical research still has not identified the exact cause(s) of Chronic Fatigue Syndrome but some research study conclusions have shown that CFS patients commonly have high blood-titers (lab result measurements) of lifetime viruses. These lifetime viruses that affect a large percentage of the population include the "Epstein-Barr virus," which causes mononucleosis in some people who contract it.

Other people are infected by the Epstein-Barr virus without symptoms but become lifetime carriers of it.

In Chronic Fatigue Syndrome patients, these viruses might explain the flu-like symptoms they experience and the swollen lymph nodes. In people with compromised immune systems, it is believed that these viruses can replicate and reactivate. This reactivation is sometimes referred-to as "post viral illness".

Co-morbid Adrenal Fatigue

It has also been found that CFS patients have less ability to cope with and recover from stress. Medical research, including that conducted by the U.S. National Institutes of Health, has found that CFS patients are low in an adrenal hormone called "cortisol." This is the "stress hormone" and studies have concluded that the low adrenal function in CFS patients might be due to an altered "hypothalamic-pituitary-adrenal axis" (HPA Axis), which is a term to describe the three endocrine glands that regulate adrenal function and work in sync with each other to supply proper levels of the cortisol hormone.

It is theorized that the function of these glands becomes "blunted" (reduced) in CFS patients, resulting in reduced adrenal cortisol levels.

Researchers do not know at this point if the low cortisol (adrenal fatigue) is a cause or a result of CFS, but they do believe it is a factor that contributes to its symptoms. A person who suspects they may have adrenal fatigue or CFS can purchase home saliva tests kits at their local pharmacy, or online, to determine if their adrenal hormones are low.

Multiple Chemical Sensitivities

In addition to the other symptoms addressed in the previous subheadings, many CFS sufferers also find that they have become sensitive to many different chemicals that they were not previously intolerant to. They may find that certain household cleaners, perfumes, deodorants, etc. cause them different types of allergic reactions or sensitivity symptoms.

This can also be true of certain foods or drinks that were not a problem before the onset of the syndrome but can be especially true of stimulants such as caffeine, chocolate and alcohol. These chemical sensitivities can trigger CFS symptoms when patients with the syndrome come in contact with them or consume them.

Neurological Symptoms

People with Chronic Fatigue Syndrome may also find that they experience headaches of a different or unusual type and/or neurological-type pain sensations. These headaches and body aches may be described as nerve-type pains and that headaches seem to radiate to other nerves within the body.

These types of nerve-related pains are sometimes referred to as "peripheral neuropathy" and can be found in other illnesses in addition to CFS, including diabetes and thyroid diseases.

Nerve-related sensations in CFS patients can include tingling and numbness in the extremities (hands and feet). Neurological symptoms can also include "Neurally Mediated Hypotension," a condition that results in blood pressure becoming irregular, especially upon first standing from a seated position, also referred to as "Orthostatic Hypotension" and "Postural Hypotension". When a CFS patient experiences this neurological symptom, they may feel dizzy and/or faint upon rising after sitting or lying down (from supine positions).

Ruling Out Other Illnesses

If other underlying medical conditions have been ruled-out as a cause of CFS symptoms, through complete and thorough blood testing and other medical lab tests, this can help point to a diagnosis of CFS.

When patients with the previously-described symptoms are thoroughly checked by their doctors and have had a complete battery of tests to rule out all possible causes, this gives a much stronger case for a diagnosis of Chronic Fatigue Syndrome.

There are many illnesses and diseases that can present with the same (or similar) symptoms of CFS but medical blood-lab tests and other diagnostic procedures that can confirm or rule out these other illnesses.

Should a patient complete such testing and be found to be "negative" for all other causes, this is the single most definitive way to confirm that a patient's symptoms are caused by CFS, rather than another underlying medical condition.

Interesting Facts about CFS

According to reputable medical sources, Chronic Fatigue Syndrome does not typically cause organ damage and is not a fatal illness, although there are disagreements and varied opinions in this regard. Studies of the syndrome have found that some patients recover from CFS within two to five years of experiencing the onset of it, while other patients may have the illness for many years or throughout their lives.

Symptom-flares of CFS can be intermittent with varied changes in the severity of them with each episode or in some patients may remain severe and ongoing.

Other interesting facts about CFS include the following:

• CFS affects over 1-million people in the U.S. alone.
• CFS is from 3 to 4 times as common in women as in men.
• CFS affects more people in their 40s and 50s than in other age groups. ---

• CFS is rare in childhood and adolescence, with teenagers being the most affected youth-group.
• CFS is more commonly referred-to as Myalgic Encephalomyelitis (ME) in the UK.

There are treatments that help to reduce the symptoms of CFS and that can help patients regain a better quality of life. Those who are diagnosed with this serious but treatable syndrome should discuss the available treatment-options with their doctors.

CHAPTER TWO

The Suspected Causes of CFS

Triggers for Chronic Fatigue Syndrome

Decades of medical research on Chronic Fatigue Syndrome has revealed a number of abnormalities in patients with the syndrome. One definitive cause has yet to be found.

Chronic Fatigue Syndrome (CFS) is a complicated and sometimes mysterious illness. Medical research studies have been ongoing for many years in attempts to find a definitive cause for the illness. Medical groups studying CFS have instead found a number of aspects of the syndrome that are clearly present but each may play a role or be one of the many factors of CFS rather than its definitive cause.

Post Viral Illness

A number of viruses studied in relation to CFS have been found to be present in significant titers (lab result measurements) in people suffering the syndrome.

Among the viruses suspected of being possible causes or triggers for CFS, are enteroviruses and retroviruses. These include the Epstein-Barr Virus (EBV) that is usually contracted during childhood and carried throughout one's lifetime, human herpesvirus 6 and the Cytomegalovirus.

Candida albican overgrowth (fungal/yeast infection), although not in the virus category has also been suspected as a possible cause or trigger for CFS.

Some of these viruses, including EBV cause no symptoms in most people when contracted (can potentially cause mononucleosis) but will increase in the number of titers found in the blood when the virus replicates.

It has been proposed as a possibility that the increased replication of viruses may occur when the immune system is not functioning well in suppressing their ability to replicate or reactivate. Reactivation would mean that a virus resurges at times, causing repeated illness in the infected person who has not fully developed immunity to it.

Imbalance in the Involuntary Nervous System

In other studies of CFS patients, they have been found to be experiencing dysfunction in their involuntary nervous systems (INS), also referred to as "autonomic failure" and "dysautonomia". The INS is responsible for regulating blood pressure with changes in physical activity and changes in positions of the body (i.e. sitting, standing and lying flat). It also regulates all other involuntary bodily functions, including respiration, digestion, kidney function, liver function, etc… and increases these functions when needed (sympathetic response) or decreases them (parasympathetic response).

An imbalance in this system will cause these functions to be inadequate at times and over-responsive at other times. If for example, physical activity is increased and blood pressure needs to rise but fails to do so, this can result in bodily fatigue due to a lack of needed blood flow to the muscles and organs of the body. If bodily functions need to decrease at times of rest or when sleep is needed but remain highly activated this will result in fatigue as well.

Dysfunction of the Immune System

Other, conclusions resulting from medical studies of CFS causes, have found that patients with the syndrome are experiencing a dysfunction of the immune system. The immunity or what might be referred to as "resistance" to viruses and allergens is greatly diminished in CFS patients. This means that the body is more susceptible to viruses and allergens and recovers more slowly from exposure and infections to them, than are people with healthy immune systems.

Infections of these types can cause a mild systemic (system-wide) inflammation in the body and cause the person experiencing them, to feel as if they are experiencing perpetual flu-like symptoms or a continual low-grade fever.

Chronic Stress

CFS patients often report in medical study questionnaires that they experienced severe, prolonged or traumatic stress, just before the onset of their CFS symptoms.

Stress is responded-to by the part of the endocrine system called the "HPA Axis", standing for the Hypothalamus-Pituitary-Adrenal gland system. When chronic stress is experienced, this system is hyper-active and over time, becomes "blunted", meaning it becomes fatigued or diminished in its ability to run at overdrive. This causes slower release of the hormones that come from these endocrine glands that work in sync (full-circle) to supply the body with stress coping abilities.

The end result of the hypothalamus stimulating the pituitary gland, which then in-turn stimulates the adrenal glands, is the release of the stress hormone "cortisol". When this system becomes blunted after extended hyperactivity, cortisol levels begin to fall or what is sometimes referred to as "hypocortisolemia" or "hypoadrenia". Some sources recognizing this mild form of adrenal dysfunction refer to it as "Adrenal Fatigue".

CHAPTER THREE

More on Dysautonomia in Chronic Fatigue Syndrome

CFS and the Involuntary Nervous System

There are many associated causes of Chronic Fatigue Syndrome but one of the more significant connections is imbalance in the involuntary nervous system - "dysautonomia".

People with Chronic Fatigue Syndrome (CFS) have been found in research studies, to be experiencing imbalances in their involuntary nervous systems (INS) or "autonomic failure". This part of the nervous system is responsible for increasing bodily functions when needed (sympathetic) and decreasing them when needed (parasympathetic). The bodily functions affected by the INS include blood pressure, heart rate, breathing, bodily fluid balance and digestion.

Imbalances in the INS also called the "autonomic nervous system" is sometimes referred to by the medical term "dysautonomia".

While strong association between dysfunction of the INS in patients with CFS has been clearly established, there is still no definitive explanation as to why this connection exists or as to whether the problems with the INS are a cause of CFS or a result of it. It is clear however that dysautonomia plays a significant role in the symptom-complex of CFS.

Orthostatic Hypotension-Dizziness upon Standing

One of the more common forms of dysautonomia experienced by CFS patients is called "Orthostatic Hypotension" (OH). This condition causes the blood pressure to drop with positional changes of the body but occurs more often when a person is rising from a seated or lying down position (supine) to a standing position. It is also referred to as "postural hypotension" and some medical sources refer to it as "neurally mediated hypotension".

Normally, blood pressure rises slightly when a person first stands up, which allows blood to be transferred from the lower part of the body, to the upper part of the body.

With orthostatic hypotension the blood pressure instead will drop slightly, causing a person to feel lightheaded, dizzy, headachey and faint. Some people with this condition do actually pass out but is not common. Because of this abnormal and sudden drop in blood pressure, some people with OH will also experience a short term increase in heart rate, referred to as "tachycardia" (beats exceeding 100 per minute without exertion). This is the body's attempt to correct the sudden episode of hypotension.

Postural Orthostatic Tachycardia Syndrome (POTS) and CFS

POTS, is a form of dysautonomia that is diagnosed by neurologists and other physicians who specialize in nervous system disorders. When symptoms of OH and tachycardia are serious enough and result in other significant symptoms, a diagnosis of POTS may be given. Some medical research groups are finding that the similarities between POTS and CFS may point to these syndromes as being one and the same in some patients, rather than being two separate illnesses.

If this is proven to be the case at some point, CFS may be placed in the category of neurological illness. While post viral illness and other proposed factors are also being studied as causes of CFS, the resulting effect on the nervous system may prove to be the most significant factor in the syndrome.

Treatments for Dysautonomia

Dysautonomia and CFS are also similar in the fact that both illnesses have no specific treatments available for them. There are effective treatments to control or to relieve symptoms of these illnesses but each patient experiences the varied symptoms of these syndromes to different degrees. Some patients may be treated with beta-blocker medications that help control blood pressure and heart rate irregularities.

Others may be treated with drugs that control neurological symptoms such as those used to treat epilepsy while others may be treated with mineral corticosteroids (mineral version of cortisolsteroid) that helps regulate blood pressure.

Yet others may be prescribed psychiatric medications to help them cope with the severity of symptoms that can impact emotions or Cognitive Behavioral Therapy that helps them cope psychologically with their syndromes.

CHAPTER FOUR

Common Symptoms and Diagnosis of Fibromyalgia

The Syndrome of Widespread and Chronic Muscle Pain

Fibromyalgia is a syndrome of widespread body pain and fatigue. There are signs and symptoms that can help to identify and diagnose fibromyalgia.

People with fibromyalgia syndrome (FMS) will find that they experience widespread and severe body pain that is chronic (ongoing). The pain will affect the muscles and joints but will also produce "tender points." These are places on the body that experience pain when pressure is applied to them, where muscles are attached to bones, at the joints.

Some in the medical community vary in their opinions as to whether FMS is a rheumatic condition or strictly a pain syndrome. Others believe it is a combination of both.

Diagnostic Criteria for Fibromyalgia

In addition to also being recognized as an inflammatory disorder, some research studies have also found that FMS may be an autoimmune-related disorder. Some medical research groups have also found that FMS and Chronic Fatigue Syndrome (CFS) have 75% crossover symptom similarities. Some published diagnostic studies have suggested that fibromyalgia is better determined when a person experiencing FMS symptoms is found to have at least 11 of the 18 possible tender points that can occur throughout the body. These are areas where pain will occur upon applying mild pressure to them, using a fingertip.

The areas on the body where these tender points may occur include the following:

• the hips
• the knees
• the back of the head near the base of the neck
• upper areas of the chest
• the upper back in the cervical spine area
• the elbows
• the shoulders

Fatigue and Sleep Disturbances

Fatigue is another major symptom of FMS and it is sometimes exacerbated by sleep disturbances that can also occur. The fatigue is often relentless and proper sleep and rest does little to alleviate it completely. Normal circadian sleep rhythms (cycles) that are supposed to occur become abnormal in fibromyalgia patients, which results in daytime sleepiness and feeling more awake during nighttime hours.

Medical research, including that conducted by the National Institutes of Health (U.S.-NIH), suggests that abnormal functioning of the adrenal glands is one possible cause of the disrupted sleep patterns, due to the adrenal hormone "cortisol" not being properly regulated by the adrenal glands in people who have fibromyalgia.

Digestive Disturbances and IBS

FMS patients may complain of severe indigestion, heartburn and acid reflux with FMS but may also experience alternating spells of constipation and diarrhea.

This may indicate that they are also suffering from Irritable Bowel Syndrome (IBS). Frequent gastritis and bloating may also manifest as part of the digestive problems that can occur with fibromyalgia.

Headaches and Sensory Disturbances

Many people with fibromyalgia experience frequent headaches and these may have a neurological aspect to them that they have not experienced previously. The headaches may sometimes have an unusual pattern to them or will affect the person's senses as they occur (i.e. eyesight, sense of smell, taste and hearing). These sensory changes can occur with headaches or may also occur without them.

These may include heightened and/or loss of sensitivity to the following:

• light
• noises
• flavors
• odors
• sense of touch

Emotional and Mental Symptoms

People with FMS may also experience symptoms of anxiety and depression and a change in mental functioning. These emotional symptoms may alternate between those of anxiety and depression or the patient may experience mostly one of these mood problems. A person with fibromyalgia may experience anxiety symptoms as an increase in chronic worry and episodes of fear, including the possibility of panic attacks. The depression may be perceived by them as a profound sadness, an emptiness or hopelessness.

This demonstrates the importance in monitoring fibromyalgia patients for any signs of worsening emotional symptoms, which may require treatment as a separate issue, in addition to treatments that are needed for rheumatic symptoms (muscle pain).

Mental functioning may also become diminished in fibromyalgia patients. They may have difficulty concentrating and will experience what is often referred to as "brain fog," a term to describe mental dullness or an inability to focus with the same sharpness they had previous to their illness.

Short-term memory loss is also experience in some FMS patients.

See Your Doctor

People who experience the symptoms described in the subheadings above need to see a qualified, licensed medial physician in order to confirm a diagnosis of fibromyalgia or other conditions with similar symptoms. Patients receiving a diagnosis of FMS can move forward with appropriate treatment, which can help to control symptoms or diminish them significantly and return them to an improved quality of life.

CHAPTER FIVE

Common Causes of Adrenal Fatigue Syndrome

Conditions that Contribute to Exhausted Adrenals

Adrenal Fatigue may be the most common health condition that exists. Chronic stressors, lack of rest and sleep and other illnesses can all be factors in this syndrome.

Some Adrenal Fatigue sources state that there are several stages of altered adrenal function that occur before the glands become exhausted. These include a stage when the glands are hyper-active or what might be referred to as the "alarm stage", followed by a "resistance stage" in which the adrenals withdraw from completing full day cycles of stress coping and finally, they reach a fatigued state in which stress-coping is greatly diminished.

If the Adrenal Fatigue stage is not treated and reversed, complete adrenal exhaustion can also be experienced.

Mental and Emotional Stressors

Ongoing chronic stress from work, school and problems in life that might arise can place added mental and emotional pressures on a person causing a draining effect on their adrenal reserves. The hormones produced by the adrenal glands will be in greater demand in these type circumstances and although they can meet that demand for reasonable periods of time, if severe and prolonged stressors continue, this ability becomes diminished over time. The main hormone affected by this syndrome is "cortisol" that supplies the body with stress-coping and recovery abilities and supplies the body with steady energy as it also aids in glucose regulation (blood sugar).

Physical Stressors

Overextending one's physical limitations over long periods of time can contribute to reduced adrenal function as well. Continually working extended shifts on a job for example that leaves a person physically exhausted would be an example of a chronic physical stressor.

Athletes that undergo strenuous training have been studied in medical research and found to experience significant, short-term increases in cortisol levels (alarm stage). Not getting proper rest to help the body recover from physical activity is also a factor in cortisol regulation.

Another example of physical stressors, are chronic diseases and illnesses that seriously affect energy levels in the body. These add physical demands on the body due to the fact that in spite of illness, people are often required to carry on the same duties and responsibilities they had before contracting their illnesses. Inflammatory diseases can be especially taxing on adrenal function because inflammation is also responded to by the cortisol hormone which is the body's natural anti-inflammatory. Cancer patients commonly experience varied degrees of adrenal insufficiency as a result of both the disease and its treatments.

Lack of Sleep

During sleep, the adrenal glands have opportunity to recharge hormone reserves.

Studies of sleep and wake cycles and their effects on adrenal hormone levels have shown that inadequate sleep can seriously affect the cortisol circadian rhythm during waking hours. An adequate number of hours for deep sleep or what is also referred to as REM-sleep (rapid eye movement stage) are required for 24 hour cortisol cycles to complete appropriately. Lack of sleep or broken sleep patterns (fragmented) can contribute to symptoms of adrenal fatigue or can be a direct cause of it. Other research studies have shown that sleep deprivation can also cause symptoms similar to those of Chronic Fatigue Syndrome and Fibromyalgia.

Excessive use of Stimulants

When a person is experiencing a lack of energy, he may resort to increased use of stimulants to get them through the day. Stimulants increase adrenal hormone levels, including adrenaline and cortisol but can also cause these hormones to drop afterward as the stimulant diminishes from the body. This can cause a vicious cycle of highs and lows and an increase in stimulant use, which can also advance to use of drugs or alcohol to cope with downward fluctuations in energy levels.

Some people become stimulant-dependent to the point of not being able to start their day without the use of one.

These scenarios occur commonly to millions of people in the U.S. and worldwide. It has in fact been suggested by some sources that adrenal fatigue may be the most common illness affecting the population in this stressful age we live in. Some statistics state that the syndrome may affect as much as 80% of the population at some point in their lives but treatments are available that help reduce symptoms and in some cases may completely resolve the illness.

CHAPTER SIX

Adrenal Fatigue or Adrenal Insufficiency?

Mild vs Full Blown Adrenal Hypofunctioning

Adrenal Fatigue is a mild form of adrenal insufficiency affecting the rhythm of the adrenal glands rather than their ability to function normally when less fatigued.

More medical doctors from all areas of practice are recognizing the syndrome known as "Adrenal Fatigue" than at any time in the past. Years of reluctance for many of them, in accepting this common stress syndrome as a real illness, came from the fact that the condition is less-than full blown adrenal insufficiency.

The diagnostic testing used to diagnose Adrenal fatigue, is often not as black and white or definitive as that used to diagnose true adrenal insufficiency. If however, it can be diagnosed, treatments are available.

Adrenal Function Testing

The test most often used to diagnose adrenal insufficient states, which are often placed in the Addison's disease category (acute adrenocortical failure) is the "ACTH Stimulation" test, also referred to as the "Cortrosyn Stimulation Test". The test is administered by injecting the testee/patient with ACTH (adrenocorticotropic hormone) which, is the hormone normally sent from the pituitary gland in the brain, to stimulate the adrenal glands to produce cortisol.

This hormone also called "cortical", is the body's stress-coping hormone that gives the body recuperative abilities to handle daily stressors and to recover from traumatic or severe stress-inducing events.

Once injected, the testee's cortisol level is monitored to see if it rises adequately, in response to being stimulated by ACTH. If the response by the adrenals is non-existent or weak, a diagnosis of adrenal insufficiency may be given as a result.

Adrenal Rhythm

With Adrenal Fatigue, the ACTH Stimulation test will usually result in a normal reading because the issue with the syndrome is not whether the adrenals can be stimulated to produce cortisol but whether they can maintain the level of cortisol in a steady rhythm as needed by the body. Adrenal Fatigue is also referred to as a condition of "low adrenal reserve", meaning the adrenals can at times function at normal or sub-normal levels but cannot complete full daily cycles of supplying cortisol to the body as it is needed. This leaves the person's body in a stressed-out state at the end of a day of coping with stressors.

At some stages of Adrenal Fatigue, cortisol can peak at times the body needs it less, such as at times of rest or sleep when less stress-coping is needed. Adversely, the cortisol reserve may become low at active times during the day when stress-coping is needed the most.

The Role of Stress in Adrenal Fatigue

One term used in describing Adrenal Fatigue, is to refer to it as a syndrome of "stressed adrenals".

The symptoms of diminished stress-coping include fatigue, nervousness, depression, irritability, the need for stimulants and a low tolerance for stressors of any kind. The syndrome often manifests in people who have experienced traumatic events (Post Traumatic Stress Disorder) or chronic stress, meaning unrelenting, prolonged and severe. It often also manifests in people with chronic diseases, including thyroid conditions, diabetes, cancer and autoimmune diseases of all types.

Adrenal Fatigue has been cited in many medical research studies, as playing a major role in conditions such as Chronic Fatigue Syndrome, Fibromyalgia and Post traumatic Stress Disorder. While the condition is not referred to as Adrenal Fatigue in these research studies, it is fully described as a condition of "mild adrenal insufficiency" and as "hypocortisolemia", among other terms.

CHAPTER SEVEN

The Accuracy of Saliva Adrenal Cortisol Testing

How does Saliva Cortisol Compare to Blood Levels?

The development of saliva test kits for measuring adrenal hormones has proven to be an accurate and convenient method of in-home testing for detecting mild forms of adrenal hypo-function.

Cortisol, the major adrenal hormone also called "cortical" is the most important hormone level tested, to determine how well the adrenal glands are functioning. Each person has two glands, each sitting directly on top of a kidney gland, located on both sides of the lower back. The glands are small, being about the size of a grape but are responsible for the body's ability to survive, cope-with and recover from stress, including everyday stressors and those that are traumatic or severe.

The adrenals also produce hormones that are precursors to sex hormones.

This means the initial hormones produced by the glands will convert into other hormones, including the sex ones, as needed in the body.

More Adrenal Testing Options are Now Available

With the emergence of recognition for mild to moderate levels of adrenal insufficiency, often referred to as "Adrenal Fatigue" or "Adrenal Exhaustion", more testing options have been developed for testing adrenal function.

In addition to the test for detecting full blown adrenal insufficiency called the "ACTH Stimulation test", other tests to detect abnormal adrenal function, including those that help detect overactive adrenal glands (Cushing's syndrome) have become increasingly available in recent years.

These tests include collecting urine samples over a 24 hour period, to determine adrenal cortisol output and saliva samples that can be collected at different times of the day to establish the rhythm of cortisol output.

Medical Research says Saliva Cortisol Tests are Accurate

Medical groups that have studied adrenal-cortisol testing by saliva samples, have determined this type testing to be accurate, as well as less intrusive and more convenient than blood sampling.

Mention is also made in these studies that multiple levels can be obtained at different points of a full day-cycle (24 hour period) which would be difficult to accomplish by blood sampling.

Saliva samples can be done in the convenience of a person's home while multiple blood draws would require long stays or repeated visits to blood draw clinics when taking multiple samples during a 24-hour period.

When citing conclusions on saliva testing to detect Cushing's syndrome, the Journal of Clinical Endocrinology & Metabolism states that it is as accurate as plasma measurements and better than urine glucocorticoid excretion.

Salivary Cortisol Measurements

Saliva Test Kits are available online and through Pharmacies. Consumers, who wish to test their adrenal function in the privacy of their homes, can now purchase saliva test kits that accurately measure both cortisol and DHEA hormone levels. Many pharmacies are now carrying kits by reputable labs that analyze saliva samples, including those manufactured by ZRT Labs, Inc. and Great Smokies Diagnostic Laboratory (GSDL). These companies also offer saliva test kits to determine sex hormone levels in addition to the adrenal ones. Saliva sex hormone testing is also used by medical research groups, including World Health Organizations.

If you order testing through your pharmacy, results are returned to them, so that your pharmacist can go over the results with you. If you order test kits online, the results are sent directly to you. While this type testing requires no doctor visit, people who use them should take their results to their doctor for evaluation if abnormal results are returned or regardless of results so that it can be entered into your medical files.

CHAPTER EIGHT

Cortisol Supplementation for Adrenal Fatigue

Are Steroids Safe for Exhausted Adrenals?

Cortisol supplementation for chronic Adrenal Fatigue carries potential risks but may be an effective treatment if administered by a qualified, monitoring physician.

People suffering chronic Adrenal Fatigue (frequent or ongoing), will often diligently seek a treatment that will provide them relief for their concerning symptoms.

For many, the option of cortisol replacement therapy is seriously considered and some patients find physicians willing to give them a trial of the treatment.

Glucocorticoids, which are synthetic cortisol replacement drugs, are steroids that require caution when used to treat adrenal disorders or health conditions of any kind.

Cortisol Supplementation Requires a Qualified Physician

While some cases of Adrenal Fatigue have been successfully treated using synthetic cortisol steroids (hydrocortisone), other cases result in further suppression of the adrenal glands by the treatment. In some cases this may be due to the dose not being monitored closely or not being dosed correctly (incorrect dose amounts). It is of most importance that this type treatment is administered by a qualified medical professional, who is knowledgeable in adrenal hormone replacement therapies. The physician would also need to be skilled in monitoring a patient's hormone levels while they are being treated. A patient considering the treatment should also be thoroughly informed about the possible risks and side effects.

Hydrocortisone Therapy in CFS Patients with low Cortisol Levels

In the year 1996, the U.S. National Institutes of Health (NIH) – Centers for Disease Control, conducted studies of Chronic Fatigue Syndrome patients.

They treated them with doses of hydrocortisone (synthetic cortisol) to replace sub-clinically low cortisol levels. The trial of cortisol replacement therapy followed other studies that found low cortsol levels in CFS patients compared to healthy controls (non-CFS participants). The study was an attempt to see if the cortisol supplementation would relieve CFS symptoms.

Over-replacing Cortisol can Cause the Adrenal Glands to Shut-down

The NIH study of cortisol supplementation in CFS patients concluded that in some of the participants, the drug significantly relieved their symptoms but an adverse effect of "adrenal suppression" (further decrease in adrenal cortical output) was seen in some of them after several weeks on the drug. This resulted in the conclusion that cortisol supplementation was not a safe treatment due to the risk of the treatment causing significant adrenal insufficiency. The outcome of the trial may have been more favorable if lower doses had been administered because CFS patients have mild adrenal insufficiency and do not require full cortisol replacement as do those with full-blown adrenal insufficiency.

Testing Cortisol Levels

With the potential risks involved in cortisol supplementation, which includes increased risk for hypertension and elevated glucose levels (high blood sugar), Adrenal Fatigue patients should consider natural methods for increasing cortisol levels safely. There are a number of potential causes for sub-clinically low adrenal function, including CFS, as addressed in the previous subheading, chronic and inflammatory diseases, traumatic stress and emotional disorders. These conditions can however first result in increased cortisol levels before causing a significant drop in them.

These facts point to the importance in first testing to determine the cortisol level before assuming it to be low and in need of being increased. If borderline low or sub-clinically low levels are not found, then boosting cortisol levels might not be what is needed. If however test results reveal the need for adrenal support, adrenal supplements may provide the needed answer. If supplements are taken to improve adrenal function, it is also important to retest adrenal hormone levels at regular intervals to monitor the treatment.

Natural Methods for Increasing Cortisol Levels

Taking safe over-the-counter supplements that help strengthen fatigued adrenal glands is recommended as a first line of treatment, rather than resorting to cortisol steroids that pose potential risks. Supplements that specifically help boost the adrenals in producing more cortisol, would be "glycyrrhizic acid" which is found in licorice root extract products and "adrenal glandular" which is found in products processed from the adrenal glands of animals.

Most adrenal glandular products are hormone free however one brand available called "Isocort" contains trace amounts of cortisol in the pellets that are processed from the adrenal glands of New Zealand sheep. It is recommended that any supplement always be taken at the manufacturer's recommended-dose and that any supplement is approved by a physician who knows a patient's medical background.

CHAPTER NINE

Effective Adrenal Fatigue Treatments

Boosting Fatigued Adrenal Glands

Adrenal Fatigue is a stress-syndrome, meaning the adrenal glands become blunted or diminished in their ability to moderate stress but there are treatments that can help.

Adrenal Fatigue, the sub-clinical form of adrenal insufficiency is not at the level of severity that full blown adrenal insufficiency is but the symptoms can still seriously affect those who develop the condition.

Following within the final subheadings in this chapter, are therapies that have been found to be effective in treating Adrenal Fatigue -- the sub-clinical type of hypoadrenia.

Proper Rest Promotes Healthy Adrenal Function

People suffering Adrenal Fatigue are typically those who push themselves too hard.

They maintain schedules that overextend their energy levels. When you combine this type of daily pace with not taking time for getting plenty of rest and proper sleep, Adrenal Fatigue can become a chronic issue. Symptoms of overextended adrenals can be improved and in some cases completely relieved by taking rest periods of a few minutes, at different points during the day. Labor laws in some areas of the world for example, require that employees are given breaks to rest and recharge their energy levels, at a rate of about 15 minutes per four hour shifts. Leisure and vacation time away from work duties is also an important aspect of getting proper rest.

Adequate Sleep can Boost the Adrenals

Getting proper sleep is also very important because studies have shown that during sleep the body repairs itself and replenishes hormone reserves that are responsible for all bodily functions and energy levels. The adrenal stress-hormone called "cortisol" is one of those hormones that requires proper sleep to maintain an adequate level of reserves.

These are needed for steady release throughout active daytime hours (circadian rhythm). Studies have also shown that the body requires 8 hours of uninterrupted sleep per 24 hour cycle. Sleep that is fragmented (interrupted) may rob the body of the deep-stages of sleep the body requires.

Reducing Stress Increases Adrenal Hormone Reserves

Chronic stress is the strongest contributing factor in the development of Adrenal Fatigue. The adrenal glands moderate stress, by releasing cortisol which helps the body cope with and recover from daily stressors. When stressors are overwhelming, traumatic or chronic, this causes hyperactive use of cortisol which over time causes reserves of the hormone to diminish due to inability of the adrenal glands to keep up with the excessive demand.

For this reason, reducing stress levels in every way possible is essential in successfully treating Adrenal Fatigue. Learning relaxation techniques, exercise routines, deep-breathing and stress reduction methods can be greatly beneficial in this area.

Eliminating Stimulants can Reduce Adrenal Stress

It is also important to remove stimulants from the diet whenever possible. Both caffeine and chocolate for example, can provide boosts in energy but afterward, an adverse drop in energy can occur. The same is true of other stimulants, including consuming moderate to large amounts of refined sugar and drinking alcohol. If stimulants are not limited or eliminated, Adrenal Fatigue sufferers may find that they experience ongoing dependency on them and a vicious cycle of highs and lows in their energy levels. It may become increasingly difficult for them to start their day without a stimulant, such as a cup of caffeinated coffee.

Adrenal Friendly Diet

A diet rich in healthy foods, including fruits, vegetables, nuts and grains (complex carbohydrates) can contribute to improved adrenal function and overall better health. Eliminating foods containing refined sugars can also be beneficial.

These types of "simple carbohydrates" supply quick-energy but afterward cause a crash and a feeling of being stressed-out as addressed earlier. Foods to avoid would be those that are manufactured and that contain refined sugars such as soft drinks, pies, cookies, cakes and candies.

Adrenal Boosting Supplements

Adding helpful over-the-counter supplements that contain adrenal-boosting properties, at the manufacturer's recommended dose can also help restore proper adrenal function. These would include vitamins B-5, B-5 and B12, with vitamin C also added which helps the B-vitamins absorb and work better in the body. Other natural supplements that have been found to help boost adrenal function and energy levels include herbals such as licorice root extract, ashwagandha, Co-Q10 enzyme, Asian Ginseng and Rhodiola Root. Beef (bovine) "adrenal glandular" which is usually hormone-free, comes from the adrenal glands of cows and processed into pill form and has also been reported to be effective in treating adrenal fatigue.

Talk to your Doctor

It is important to fully inform your doctor about any supplements you may choose to take, so that he can determine whether or not they are safe in adding them to any treatments you are currently undergoing. Monitoring for any unpleasant or concerning side effects is also important when adding a supplement of any kind to your treatment regimen.

CHAPTER TEN

Diagnosing and Treating Addison's Disease

Symptoms of Autoimmune Adrenalitis

While there are other types of adrenal insufficiency that fall under the category of "Addison's disease", the most common type is autoimmune adrenalitis. This type of adrenal dysfunction is full-blown, rather than mild as is experienced with Adrenal Fatigue. It is important that people, who believe they are experiencing true adrenal hypo-function rather than a milder form of Adrenal Fatigue, are properly tested by medical lab analysis.

Addison's disease is most commonly an autoimmune disorder affecting the adrenal glands. Each person has two adrenal glands, which are part of the endocrine system (hormone producing) and they sit on top of each kidney in a person's body. These glands are small and shaped like pyramids about the size of a walnut, measuring about 3 x 5 x 1 cm in size.

The immune system can mistakenly recognized these glands as intruders and begin to attack them (autoimmune response), slowly destroying them with auto-antibodies (killer cells from the immune system). This is the most common cause of Addison's disease.

Addison's Disease Results in Hormone Deficiency

When the onset of Addison's disease occurs, this causes the adrenal glands to become inadequate in supplying the important adrenal hormones needed by the body, the two major hormones being "cortisol" and "DHEA" (dehydroepiandrosterone). Symptoms of Addison's disease appear once at least 90% of the adrenal cortex (the protective outer layer of the gland) has been destroyed by the autoimmune process known as "autoimmune adrenalitis".

Addison's Disease Symptoms

The symptoms of Addison's disease are those of adrenal hormone deficiency. Addison's disease causes adrenal insufficiency, meaning a reduction in adrenal hormone production and output.

The two major hormones that become low due to this disease process are cortisol and DHEA.

Cortisol is the "stress hormone" and "anti-inflammatory hormone" that gives the body its ability to handle and recover from stressors and inflammation. DHEA is a "sex hormone precursor", meaning the hormone that converts into testosterone, estrogen and other male and female sex hormones needed by the body.

When the adrenal hormones become low, a person may experience the following symptoms of low adrenal function.

• fatigue
• joint/muscle pain
• weight loss
• diminished appetite
• low blood pressure (hypotension)
• hyper-pigmentation (darkening of the skin)

If left untreated, people with Addison's disease are at risk of experiencing an adrenal crisis, meaning they can potentially go into shock and possibly coma or death.

Diagnosing Addison's Disease

Addison's disease is most often diagnosed through blood testing and MRI (magnetic resonance imaging). Medical blood lab testing can measure the adrenal hormone levels and if they are found to be low, this can indicate adrenal insufficiency due to Addison's disease.

Patients will then usually be tested for adrenal function via an ACTH Stimulation Test. This test uses the ACTH hormone, which usually comes naturally from a person's own pituitary gland, to stimulate adrenal-cortisol hormone production but, during the test, it is administered to the patient by injection.

A patient will have a baseline blood draw taken before the test. After the ACTH hormone injection, they will have two or more additional blood draws taken at 30 minute intervals, and these three blood levels will then be compared. If the two or more additional blood levels of cortisol do not significantly increase above the baseline level, a diagnosis of adrenal insufficiency is confirmed.

Other tests that may be ordered would include an MRI to detect the extent of adrenal gland destruction, and a blood test to detect antibodies that the immune system is directing against the adrenal glands.

Treatment for Addison's Disease

Addison's disease is treated by replacing the low adrenal hormone levels. Once blood tests reveal which adrenal hormones are low, hormone replacement therapy will begin. One of the major hormones called cortisol, which is most commonly low in adrenal insufficiency states, must be replaced with a steroid cortisol substitute called a "corticosteroid" also referred to as "hydrocortisone". Patients will need replacement with this synthetic hormone and any others found to be low, for the rest of their lives.

Addison's disease patients are also usually required to wear a medical ID bracelet, so that if they experience an adrenal crisis (sudden, severe drop in adrenal hormones), the person finding them will know that they are treated for Addison's disease.

It may also indicate that, they need to have an emergency-dose of corticosteroid steroid administered by a doctor.

There are a number of other causes of adrenal insufficiency, but Addison's disease is the most common, affecting about 1 in 100,000 people according to medical sources. Anyone who suspects they may be experiencing symptoms of adrenal insufficiency should see their doctor for immediate evaluation.

CHAPTER ELEVEN

How to Set Reasonable Health Goals

Resolving to Become Healthier

Most everyone has resolved at different times in their lives to live healthier through improved diet and exercise. Improving one's overall fitness is a wise resolution and is especially important for those who suffer health problems such as CFS, Fbromyalgia and/or Adrenal Fatigue.

Goals for becoming healthier are better achieved if they are reasonably set, with expectations being attainable rather than a near-impossibility to reach.

Gradual improvements in diet, exercise and stress-reduction are those that are more easily attained and that are more successfully held onto and improved upon. Methods for pacing one's self to accomplish health resolutions at a successful pace will be addressed in the subheadings that follow.

Common Health Resolutions

Goals for better health are often referred to as "resolutions" and many people set them within days or weeks before the change of a new year. The following are goals that people making resolutions commonly desire improvement-in, for overall better health.

• weight loss
• a healthier, low-fat diet
• exercising to tone the body and improve stamina
• a plan for dealing-with and reducing stress

Many people have found through trial and error, that setting reasonable goals rather than ones that are very difficult to achieve, helps one to remain inspired to achieve them, rather than becoming discouraged before reasonable gains are made.

Improved Diet and Weight Loss

When improving one's diet for weight loss, the goal should also include the improvement of health. This would mean to not only eat less but to eat healthier foods as well.

Starvation diets, for example, are not healthy and can result in a person binge-eating once they see weight loss resulting and they are tempted to compromise their diet. Gradual weight loss has been shown in studies to be healthier and weight that is more easily kept-off, rather than regained.

Cutting out fattening foods by what is sometimes called the "cold turkey" method, in which they are stopped suddenly and completely may also be less successful for some dieters than a more gradual cutting-out of fatty foods. If a person resolves to completely remove white and sweet breads from their diet, for example, they might better achieve this by eating 50% less white bread at first and then cutting it back another 25% over a few weeks time and weaning off the last 25% within a few more weeks.

Unhealthy foods should also be replaced with healthy ones, to include vegetables, fruits, nuts and grains.

Reasonable Exercise Routines

Exercise is quite possibly the single healthiest pursuit one can undertake.

Studies have shown that it not only improves muscular tone in the body and cardiovascular health but it can also improve one's emotions and help to reduce stress levels.

Whether one begins an aerobics or calisthenics exercise regimen, they should do so at a pace their bodies can tolerate well. Extending beyond one's tolerance level can result in bodily injury and unnecessary fatigue. By beginning a low-impact and safe level of exercise, one can gradually build the level as they are able to safely adjust to it.

Walking is a safe way to begin a cardiovascular, aerobics exercise routine, building speed and distance at a gradual pace. Low repetition calisthenics, using no weights, then slowly graduating to light weights and heavier weights can be a safe method for a body toning routine.

Reducing Stress

No one is immune to the effects of stress in everyday life but it can be reduced and maintained at a healthier level through stress-reduction practices.

This area of improvement for better health takes time and effort to achieve but can contribute both to improved physical and emotional well-being.

As mentioned in the previous subheading, exercise is a great natural stress-reducer. Other methods for reducing and gaining control over stress include enjoyable pastimes and hobbies such as art pursuits and leisure activities. The following are hobbies and leisure activities that can be enjoyed while reducing stress levels.

• writing
• painting
• sculpting
• hiking
• camping
• games
• music
• reading

Taking time out to simply rest quietly or to meditate can also contribute to stress reduction. These activities can have a cumulative effect toward conquering stressors that exert negative effects on mental and physical health.

In conclusion, it is wise when making resolutions for better health, to include all three areas of improvement as addressed in the previous subheadings. Each of these can contribute to the success of the others for a well-balanced improvement in overall health.

CHAPTER TWELVE

When is DHEA Supplementation Beneficial?

The Non-prescription Adrenal Hormone Treatment

With some adrenal insufficient states, it is the DHEA hormone that is deficient but under what conditions is it safe to replace the low hormone via supplementation?

DHEA is an essential adrenal hormone that carries out a number of important purposes in the body. The hormone can become low due to certain types of disease processes, such as autoimmune, inflammatory and chronic health disorders but also decreases in the body with age.

Levels of DHEA can drop below normal values or remain in a low-normal state, which may require hormone replacement therapy. When DHEA is supplemented when it is not needed, it can cause adverse effects in the body.

What is DHEA?

The full medical name for this hormone is "dehydroepiandrosterone" and is a hormone that is endogenous, meaning it is made in the human body, even though it can be supplied to the body from an outside source. Being the most abundant adrenal hormone in the body, it is manufactured by the adrenal glands and afterward is converted into other essential hormones, as they are needed. It is also referred to as a steroid but because it undergoes a synthesizing process in the brain, it is also called a neurosteroid.

DHEA is available over-the-counter in supplement form and most brands are made from extracts derived from wild Mexican yams. Claims by some medical sources and by research done by firms that manufacture DHEA supplements, the hormone can increase positive mood, sex drive, immune system function and energy levels when supplemented. It is important to add that these benefits would only be realized if supplementation with the hormone is done so at the dose needed and at a level that does not adversely affect sex hormone balance.

Precurser to Sex Hormones

A major function of DHEA is converting into sex
hormones for both males and females. All sex
hormones are common to both sexes but in
different balance for each gender. The male
hormones DHEA converts into are referred to as
androgens and the female hormones it converts
into are referred to as estrogens. Because of the
hormone being available to convert into these
other hormones this also places it in the category
of being a "precursor hormone", meaning it is on
stand-by to convert as needed.

Hyperandrogenism in Men and Women

It is important that DHEA levels are in proper
balance in women, due to the risk of too many
male hormones being produced through
conversion if levels become too high. The term
for too much male hormone production is
"hyperandrogenism" and can result in a condition
called hirsutism in women, in which there is
excessive growth of body hair. Other symptoms
of hyperandrogenism in women can include acne,
increased muscle growth, changes in sex drive,
decreased breast size and a deeper voice tone.

67

Some medical sources state that about 10% of the female population is experiencing some degree of hirsutism from hyperandrogenism.

A major cause of hyperandrogenism in women is "polycystic ovary syndrome" (PECOS) in which the ovaries cause an excessive amount of androgens to be produced.

It can also be caused by overproduction of DHEA from the adrenal glands, from over-supplementing with DHEA or from taking doses of the hormone when it is not needed.

Hyperandrogenism can also occur in males but symptoms and manifestations of the condition are less noticeable in adult males. When symptoms do occur, they can include male pattern baldness (alopecia), acne, abnormally high testosterone levels, changes in sex drive and irritability.

In pre-teen males, hyperandrogenism can cause early onset and an abnormal increase in the advancement of puberty.

Testing Before Supplementing

With the risk of inducing hyperandrogenism from supplementing with DHEA when there is not a need for it, this points to the great importance in first testing the hormone's level before attempting to increase it in the body. Adrenal hormone testing usually includes both the DHEA and cortisol levels because these hormones interact with each other, creating a ratio between them. According to some medical sources, DHEA can suppress cortisol levels and vise-versa and supplementing one may also require supplementing the other to keep the ratio balanced.

Opinions vary as to what a safe supplemented amount of DHEA would be. Some sources state that up to 25mg in females and up to 50mg in males is a safe dose however, this would not be the case if DHEA levels are already at proper-normal, high-normal or flagged-high. Supplementation added at these levels, could cause adverse side effects as previously described and demonstrates the importance in testing adrenal and sex hormone levels before considering supplementation.

A patient can test hormone levels and supplement with DHEA on his own if levels are low but should do so with extreme caution, making sure to retest the hormone levels at regular intervals to monitor the treatment. The better and safer scenario would be to have a treating doctor order saliva and/or blood-serum adrenal and sex hormone tests, to assure that DHEA supplementation is safe for a patient and so that he can determine the proper dosage needed.

(END)

About the Author:

I am a husband, father, grandfather and lifetime contract salesman, with experience in health writing that began in 2004. I completed theological studies with Liberty University in 1996. I formerly served as editor and forum moderator of Thyroid Health for a major multi-topic content site and as a general health writer for another, where I received Editor's Choice Awards for my articles on health subjects. In 2003 I was diagnosed with hypothyroidism; "Hashimoto's thyroiditis" being the cause. This autoimmune form of thyroid disease that causes destruction of the thyroid gland resulted in my also developing "Chronic Fatigue Syndrome", due to a compromised immune system with severe co-morbid "Adrenal Fatigue". I also suffered severe anxiety symptoms, including panic attacks early into the onset of Hashimoto's thyroiditis (Hashitoxicosis). I was also diagnosed with peripheral neuropathy and thyroid myopathy, with co-morbid nutritional deficiencies. My eventual receiving of diagnoses was a difficult process with proper diagnostic testing not being ordered by the first doctors I sought treatment from. These types of issues were inspiration for me to become proactive in my own health care and to self-educate myself on these health disorders, which I have done extensively since 2003. I now enjoy sharing this information with other patients experiencing my same health disorders.

(END)

The Best Darn CFS, Fibromyalgia and Adrenal Fatigue Book!

www.ingramcontent.com/pod-product-compliance
Lightning Source LLC
Chambersburg PA
CBHW071327310526
45789CB00016B/1257